# I Believe in Miracles

# I Believe in Miracles

A Conversion Journey

Lourdes W. Arriola

**To order additional copies of this book, contact:**
Xlibris Corporation
1-888-795-4274
www.Xlibris.com
Orders@Xlibris.com
74844

# CONTENTS

# Prologue

All my life, I have never found it easy to share my innermost thoughts and feelings with others. I have never been one to stand up in front of a group, to give voice to my thoughts or my opinions, even when I had very strong feelings about the issue. A friend once said that I was much too inhibited. I have no doubts he was right. There were certainly occasions when I wanted very much, to share with some people, my feelings, my thoughts, but something inside me kept me from doing so. I can remember at least a couple of occasions when this happened. I remember at my daughter's wedding, how I had wanted very much to tell the guests and our new son-in-law, how my husband and I were so happy to welcome him to our family. I had even written a little speech about the first time we met him.

About a year or so before the wedding, my daughter, who at that time was in school in Germany, called to tell us that she had seen a doctor there because of a lump in her neck. He biopsied it, and told her she had metastatic cancer. That was the most devastating news I had ever heard! She was only 26 years old. She had just recently graduated from Law School. With a background degree in Electrical Engineering, she had decided to go to Germany to specialize in Intellectual Property Law. My husband and I were very happy for her, thinking she was going to have a wonderful life ahead of her. Now it seemed it was not to be. Instead her life was going to be cut short. I told her I wanted her to come home. I didn't want a doctor I didn't even know, treating her. While we were talking, I was already mentally figuring how my husband would have to go to Germany to pick her up. I certainly did not want her sitting on that plane, alone for 8 hours, thinking of her diagnosis. Then a male voice came over the phone, introduced himself as her friend, and asked if it was alright with us for him to accompany her on the trip home. In my mind, I was thinking I would be eternally grateful to him, but true to my inhibited nature, I just said it would be alright. We met them at the airport two days later. That was the first time we met Michael.

That week was a roller coaster of emotions. Initially, a friend of mine who was a pathologist looked at the biopsy slides, and said it didn't look like cancer. We were so happy! We celebrated with a lunch at a nice restaurant. Then in the afternoon, she called to tell me she had shown the slides to another pathologist, one who was internationally known as an expert in fine needle biopsies and she said it was malignant. It threw us into a tailspin! We were told we needed to see a thyroid specialist. A thyroid specialist I knew personally, was kind enough to accommodate us that afternoon. Although he could not tell from examining her, if she had a thyroid problem, he suggested that we see a thyroid surgeon, because of the opinion given by the pathologist on the basis of the biopsy slides. We made an appointment to see a thyroid surgeon the next day. The thyroid surgeon we consulted did not agree with her diagnosis. He felt sure on the basis of his examination that it was just an aberrant salivary tissue, however, because he was contradicting the opinion of a widely respected pathologist, he needed to do a biopsy of the lump. Fortunately, the biopsy proved that he was right. Thank God, he was right and she was wrong. As horrible as that week was, my husband and I agreed one good thing had come out of it. We got to meet her boyfriend, saw how very much he loved her, and how protective he was of her. We told ourselves, that if they ever came to tell us they wanted to get married, we would give them our blessings, no questions asked. We had no doubts that he was the right man for her and we would be very happy to welcome him to our family. Well, I had the speech prepared, but in the end, I opted not to say anything.

Another occasion when I kept silent when I should have spoken was when a very good friend of ours died. This was a man, whose friendship my husband and I treasured. At the wake, when we were asked to share our memories of him, I wanted very much to tell everyone what a special person he was! I could have shared with those who did not know him well, what a kind, compassionate, and caring person he was. I could have told them stories about his wonderful sense of humor. Or I could even have told them about his homemade pizza and his delicious hamburgers that my children loved to eat during cookouts at their house. Again, I decided to say nothing. I have since regretted not giving voice to my thoughts, on both those occasions and others as well. Yet through the years, I continued to be very "protective" of my innermost thoughts and feelings, unwilling, or unable to share them with others.

Then during a retreat I attended a few years ago, I heard the story of a pair of ants. The story goes, a couple of ants were walking on a tabletop when they spotted a chocolate bar. They tasted it. They said this is so delicious, we simply have to share it with our family! Then the entire family said this is so delicious, we must share it with our friends. So before you knew it, the chocolate bar was entirely covered with ants feasting on it, and thoroughly enjoying the experience. The moral of the story, according to the retreat master, was that sometimes, something happens in our lives, that is "so delicious" that our whole being cries out to share it with others.

Well, in 2003, something happened in my life which at first blush seemed like a total tragedy. As a matter of fact, that was exactly the way I thought of it initially. But then gradually, I was led on a journey that would completely change my life! A conversion journey that has brought me unprecedented joy. Indeed, the experience has been "so delicious" that I have decided to share it with whoever might feel so inclined to listen. Hence, this book.

# Chapter 1

# A life-changing Diagnosis

One beautiful Spring morning in June 2003, something happened that completely changed my life. When I got up that morning, I had no idea that my life was going to be altered forever. As I went through my morning routine; shower, getting dressed, putting on my make-up, my mind was preoccupied with my plans for the day. I was going to have my mammogram at St Joseph Hospital, after which I planned to spend the rest of the day scouring for plants at Frank's gardens, Home Depot, and Lowe's. For the past two months, I had been very busy putting in two gardens, a rose garden in the back of the house, and an eclectic one in the front. All my days off from my practice were spent on these projects. As I got myself ready for my appointment, in my mind, the mammogram was just a necessary nuisance I had to deal with, before I could really enjoy the rest of the day. My husband was sitting at his computer desk when I told him "bye, see you when I see you" which meant don't bother waiting up for me for lunch, thinking I would probably be gone the whole day. According to a friend of mine, my problem is, I am such a cheapskate that I would spend hours in the "intensive care units" of Home Depot and Lowe's, just to find bargains. Invariably, I would end up with some half dead plants that would need a lot of TLC, to get them to flourish. In her mind, that was wasting a lot of time just to save a little money. True, my forays into what we called the "intensive care units" of the nurseries entailed a lot of time, but I thoroughly enjoyed these expeditions! To me, picking up a plant that was practically dead, for practically nothing, and then nursing it to life and seeing it bloom, was worth all the time and energies I put into it. I looked at this as a genetic predisposition. My mother was such an avid gardener. As a child growing up in the Philippines, I was used to seeing my mother spend a lot of her time nurturing her plants. She had an uncanny knack for nursing sorry looking plants into gorgeous bloomers. Growing up, I never showed any interest in all these endeavors of my mother, so I was pleasantly surprised, when as I got older, I became enthralled with the idea of having my own garden. In some ways, it made me feel connected to my mother. As I drove to the hospital that morning, my mind was already busy at work imagining the rest of that morning and afternoon, when I would be at the nurseries, happily looking for the plants I wanted for my gardens.

When I got to the Hospital, two things happened that I had not expected. First, when I started to fill up the forms, I found out I had missed 2 mammograms instead of one. I thought it had been a year and a half since my last mammogram, but their records showed that it actually had been two and a half years. I guess I had been so busy I had not noticed the passing of time. This was ironic, because in my practice, I was always very adamant that my patients did their yearly mammograms. Excuses like, "but they are so painful" would elicit from me the response, "a little pain won't kill you, but breast cancer will, if you don't discover it early." That I would have been so careless with my own health was beyond me. Being busy was not an acceptable excuse in my mind. Then when the young technician came into the room, she asked me if this was a routine exam or if I had a mass. I had been going to this hospital for my mammograms for over twenty years and nobody had ever asked me that question! In my mind, this was just a routine mammogram and I don't know why I said I do have a very small mass. Actually, the mass I was talking about had been there for as many years and they had been reading my yearly mammograms as normal but densely fibrocystic, so I was convinced that it was just a cyst. On top of that, through all those years, the mass had never changed in size or consistency. Also, I had exactly the same size mass in the same location on the other breast. I figured these were just part of the cystic elements in my breasts, thinking that the chances of them being cysts were more likely than having cancer in both breasts. It should be noted at this point however, that it is possible to have multiple sites of cancer in both breasts, not often, but can happen nevertheless. At any rate, she said that a mass automatically necessitated an ultrasound. I said fine, and we went on with the exam. In retrospect, if I could do it over again, I would have insisted on having an ultrasound with my mammograms, knowing that a small mass could be missed in the case of a dense fibrocystic breast, instead of presuming that it was a cyst, because the mammograms were read as negative. When we were finished, the technician left the room, presumably to show the films to the radiologist before letting me go.

When the technician came back to the room, another young woman came in with her, introducing herself to me as the radiologist. She asked if she could examine me. She looked very concerned. Fear was now gripping me. I asked her what the problem was. She said there was a "very slight change" in my mammogram and the ultrasound showed some enlarged nodes in my axilla (the armpit). Being a physician, I knew the significance of enlarged axillary nodes. It did not augur well. I tried to hold back the tears, as I listened to her telling me about a very good breast surgeon in the hospital. I thanked her, and got out of there as fast as I could. In the privacy of my car, I let loose the flood of tears. Oddly, just a week before, I had the sad task of telling a patient that she had metastatic cancer of the lung. For years, I had been trying to get this patient to stop smoking, but her answer was always the same. She loved smoking, so she would not quit. She would just deal with whatever would happen in the future. Well, after not seeing her for about a year and a half, she came in to the office with a few lumps in her neck. I knew as soon as I saw them, that this was what I had dreaded all along, and of course the Ct scan of the chest proved it. When I talked to her about the findings of the CT scan confirming the diagnosis of lung cancer, she sat there stoically, listening to me without showing any emotion, while her husband had tears in his eyes. After they left the office, with the promise that she would make an appointment with the oncologist as soon as possible, I sat at my desk for a while. I wondered what she was truly feeling inside. I wondered how it felt to be told you have cancer. Well now I knew! I felt as though my whole world was imploding!

For the past several years, my husband and I had been enjoying the "good life." The kids had all graduated from college, and were having good lives of their own. My husband and I were relishing the freedom of being able to go anywhere, anytime we pleased. I had a busy practice that I enjoyed very much and for the past two years I had been giving vent to my gardening passion and loving it! I had so much energy and so much "joie de vivre", I had no inkling, that something so malevolent was growing in my body! As I sat in my car in the Hospital parking lot, I had the gut wrenching feeling, that this was the end of the "beautiful life" I had been living. Now I was faced with so much uncertainty. With the knowledge that there were some enlarged lymph nodes in my axilla, it was obvious to me, that the cancer had already escaped from the breast. To me, that meant my chances of cure were not so great. The memory of patients and friends, who had died of this dreaded disease, flashed through my mind. I thought of my husband, my children, and my grandchildren. I wondered how much time I would have left to enjoy them. My heart felt so heavy! I don't know how long I sat there crying, feeling so sad at the thought that we might not have much time. After a while, I decided I needed to compose myself. I had the difficult task ahead, of telling my husband the bad news. While I was driving home, I debated different ways to break the news to my husband. Should I tell it to him straight, or should I soft pedal it, so as not to scare him. My husband is not a physician, so I figured he would take the cue from me. If I did not seem worried, then he would most likely think there was not much to worry about. I decided I would just tell him that I had an abnormal mammogram, and that I needed to see the breast surgeon. No need to upset him. When I walked into the bedroom, my husband was still at his computer desk. He looked quizzically at me, obviously not expecting me to be home so soon. I burst into tears, completely forgetting my resolve to keep my composure. He held me tightly, while I cried like a baby!

The next few days were a blur. I made the appointment with the surgeon, we stocked the refrigerator with a lot of antioxidant foods, read books on macrobiotic diets, sort of closing the barn door after the horse was gone. The question now, was how to tell the kids and when. Father's day was about a week away, so we decided to wait. We knew we had to tell them at some point, but we figured it was better for them to be spared of the bad news even for just a few more days. They would be calling their dad to wish him a happy father's day, so we would just tell them then. After talking to the kids, I got busy with the usual work-up prior to surgery. It is called staging, trying to see what stage I was in, so as to decide if I was a candidate for surgery. I had a lot of blood work, Ct of the chest and abdomen, and bone and brain scans. Thank God, the tests showed no distant metastases. That meant the cancer cells had not gone to the other organs of my body yet. At this point, it was considered to be confined to the breast and the axilla. I would have surgery followed by chemotherapy and radiation.

The surgery was actually easy. I had a modified radical mastectomy with lymph node dissection. I woke up from the general anesthesia without any side effects. I did not even take the pain pills that they offered me. I had no need for them. I was out of the hospital in 2 days. Physically, I was fine. I think I was just very glad to get rid of the offending breast! I thought of it as the 'enemy', and the sooner I got rid of it the better. Emotionally however, I was a basket case. The surgeon had come in to my room as soon as I woke up from the anesthetic, to tell me that I had 17 positive lymph nodes! That was devastating news! I had not expected to have that many. I had hoped for maybe 3 or 4. Then a few days later, when I finally had the courage to look at my pathology report, it was even more devastating. It showed that some of the lymph nodes were matted, which meant to me, that some of the cancer cells had probably gotten out of the confines of the lymph nodes. I could just imagine them floating in my bloodstream, seeding distant organs like my liver and my lungs, producing little nests of cancer cells which were still too small to be detected by the Ct scans. My official diagnosis was Breast cancer stage 3 C, but in my mind, I wondered if I was actually stage 4. I remember thinking, "you're in big trouble Lourdes." I had never felt so hopeless and so helpless in my entire life! I felt as though I was standing on the edge of a precipice, looking down into a dark bottomless abyss. I sat there on my bedroom floor with the report in my hand, tears streaming down my face, and I remember saying over and over again, "Please, Lord hold me, hold me, do not let me fall." I think it was at that moment, that I decided I would not trust myself to just chemotherapy and radiation. Sure, I would go through whatever the oncologist wanted me to do, but I had to go to a Higher Power for help with the healing I needed. Fortunately for me, I knew exactly how to go about it.

All my life, whenever I needed favors from God, big or small, I would always go through the Blessed Mother. I thought of her as the most powerful intercessor, for how could Jesus say no to His mother! I always had in mind, that the first miracle Jesus did, the changing of the water into wine, at the wedding in Cana, was the result of a subtle request from the Blessed Mother. Growing up, I had always felt a special claim to the Blessed mother's affections. After all, my relationship with her had been forged way before I was born. The story goes, my mother had 3 boys before me. Afraid that she would never have a daughter, when she found out she was pregnant for the fourth time, she made a novena to the Blessed Mother. She asked for a girl. She promised that if the baby was a girl, she would name her Lourdes, in honor of the Blessed Virgin of Lourdes and she would teach her the devotion to the Blessed Mother. Apparently, when I was born, my grandfather had wanted to name me Georgia, his sister's name, but my mother who was ordinarily quite docile and hated confrontations, stood her ground. She was not going to break her promise to the Blessed Mother. The Blessed Mother had been kind enough to give her a daughter and she would honor her, by naming her only daughter after her. The funny thing is, my mother went on to have 8 more kids, 6 boys and 2 more girls, but that's another story. Anyway, all through my childhood, she made sure I prayed the 3 Hail Marys before I went to sleep every night, and on Sundays when we went to church she dressed me up in white with a blue sash. So all my life, I have never been able to sleep at night, without praying my 3 Hail Marys. However, I stopped wearing the white dress and blue sash in High school. One of the nuns told me in no uncertain terms, that it did not go with our official Sunday gala uniform and would not be tolerated. As I said, anytime I needed anything from God, I always went through the Blessed Mother, and as far as I could remember she had never disappointed me. This time however, the stakes had never been higher and she and I had our work cut out for us. I was never without my rosary, especially during my chemotherapy sessions. I wanted to make sure she was always there with me. Whenever I had to go through a Ct scan or an MRI, I never felt the need for an anti-anxiety agent such as Xanax, which many patients use to overcome the claustrophobia, which comes with being put through these machines. As soon as I lay down on the table, I would close my eyes and pray my rosary. I would only open them again, when the technician would inform me that the test was over and I could get off the table.

# Chapter 2

# The Ordeal

I started chemotherapy about 2 or 3 weeks after surgery. I had decided to go to the University of Michigan. My daughter Trinnie, who had gone with me to my consultations with 3 different Oncologists, thought it best for me to go there, since she felt that they were in the forefront of cancer research. She figured that would enable me to avail myself of any new advances in the research of breast cancer. About 6 months before my diagnosis, a study from Sloan Kettering showed somewhat better results in the survival rate of breast cancer patients with axillary adenopathy by using a dose densed protocol. It meant giving the chemotherapy every 2 weeks instead of the standard 3 week regimen. The idea was, by giving it at shorter intervals, the cancer cells would not have as much time to multiply. There would be no respite for the cancer cells from the poisonous chemicals. However, this method not only wrought havoc to the cancer cells, but they also did the same damage to the normal cells, especially the rapidly multiplying cells such as the lining of the Respiratory and the Gastrointestinal tract and the Bone Marrow.

My regimen initially consisted of 4 cycles of Adriamycin and Cytoxan given every 2 weeks. While the surgery had been a breeze, the chemotherapy was very difficult. My normal cells were suffering just as badly as we hoped the cancer cells would. As expected, I lost all my hair, my eyebrows, and my lashes. These were some of the expected side effects of chemotherapy, so I knew they would happen at some point, but looking down at globs of my hair, in my hands, when I shampooed, was very disconcerting. I think this is why some cancer patients decide to shave their heads before starting chemotherapy, so they would not have to go through the emotionally painful experience of going bald slowly, picking up handful of hairs from the bathroom floor after a shower, or finding a lot of hair on the pillowcase, on waking up in the morning. As I have said before, when I had the mastectomy, I really did not mourn the loss of my breast, if anything, I was glad to get rid of it. It was the 'enemy'. But losing my hair was emotionally painful, because I considered them as just the innocent victims of the war between the cancer cells and the chemo drugs. My hair had never been my "crowning glory", as a matter of fact, I used to complain a lot about my hair having no distinct character; it was neither black nor brown, it was straight, it was limp, had no "body" to speak of, and yet, as I picked handsful of them from the sink or the floor, I could not help feeling the pain of losing a part of me. Sometimes, I would not succeed in stemming the tears. I had to keep reminding myself, that someday, my hair would grow back again. Sometimes, facetiously, I would console myself with the idea, that maybe, just maybe, when my hair grew back, I would have thick jet-black curly hair, like my cousin Pearl's, that I had been so envious of, when I was 10 years old. Soon after I had lost all my hair, my fingernails and my toenails started becoming discolored and they too fell off. There was no physical pain involved in all of these, just a lot of sadness, so I kept telling myself that this meant the cancer cells were being destroyed too.

The effects on my Gastrointestinal and Respiratory tracts were something else. My mouth and my tongue were full of sores which made talking difficult and eating even more so. On top of that, my taste buds must have been affected too, because I had no taste for anything. Everything tasted like paper and I had no appetite. I lost a total of 28 lbs. I would wake up in the morning with swollen, bleeding eyes and nose. It would take me several minutes before I could pry my eyes open. Quite a few times, I had so much pain in my stomach, unrelieved by ordinary pain pills (I refused to use narcotics). Those were the times, when I thought the idea of dying might not be so bad after all. Those were the times, when I would say in my most exasperated voice, "God why don't we just get this over with? Why don't You just let me die right now?" Thank God for Alberto, who was always there to bring me back to sanity. He would say, "Des, isn't it enough that you are so dramatic with me? Must you do that with God too?" Alberto had always said, I have this melodramatic streak in me, which would come to the fore whenever I was on the losing end of an argument. He should know! He has been married to me for over forty years! At any rate, his joking remark would remind me, that my mother, God rest her soul, would have been very unhappy with that kind of behavior from me. I could almost hear her again saying, "do not ever, ever be disrespectful to God!" So my little tantrum would end up with me saying in my mind, "I am so sorry mama." I should probably have said sorry to God too, because He was actually the One I was disrespecting, but I suppose I just figured He would understand. It was funny though, that as bad as I felt, I never even thought of skipping my scheduled chemo. My oncologist, knowing how miserable I felt, would say to me, "the cancer cells are very unhappy right now," and I would say "I don't want them unhappy, I want them dead."

As difficult as my first 4 cycles of chemotherapy was, I had no idea that the next months would even be worse. The next course, was for me to take Taxol. I was actually not very happy with the idea. I had wanted Taxotere ( the other taxane) which from my readings, seemed to me, to be more powerful than the taxol. I wanted the most powerful drug they could use to hit the cancer cells. However, the protocol they were using at the University had taxol as the second drug and I had no choice in it. So I started with my first dose of the Taxol. Everything was fine until about a couple of days later. I developed high fever, which necessitated my hospitalization at St Joes. They could not find out what was wrong with me and after a few days, my oncologist told me to just get out of the hospital, afraid I might catch an infection there. Instead, she would see me as an outpatient at U of M in a few days. While waiting for my appointment, I had fever and night-sweats so terrible, I had to change my bedclothes 3-4 times at night, because I would be soaking wet. Thank God, Veronica, my younger daughter, had come home from New York to help us. I was so weakened by the siege that I needed help to change my pajamas and to take my medications.

When I finally saw my oncologist, she was very hesitant to give me any more taxane because of my severe reaction to the Taxol. She had me see the Pulmonary specialist, and in the meantime, I would be off chemotherapy until she could decide what to do. For three weeks, I was in Limbo! Those three weeks of not knowing what could be done were very difficult for me. I could sense that my oncologist was not keen on continuing me on the taxane, but a friend of mine, who was an oncologist too, was very adamant that I should get the complete course of the Taxane. He even offered to give it to me himself, if nobody else wanted to. He said that was my only chance of surviving the disease. But I was hesitant to take him up on his offer. I was afraid that if I happened to die as a reaction to the Taxane that he would give me, he would feel very guilty. So I decided to wait for my oncologist's decision. I spent that time reviewing the literature on reactions to the Taxanes and I gathered that it was not very common but certainly fatal in most cases. In my search of the literature, I was able to find only 12 cases. Most of the reports consisted of only 2 or 3 patients. The biggest study had 4 patients. In all the cases I reviewed, everyone died except one. I kept saying to God, "why did You let this happen to me? Now my chance of surviving this disease is completely nil, since my oncologist will not give me the Taxane anymore." Needless to say, I was very unhappy with Him at that time, not realizing then, that one day, I would know the reason for all this, and I would be very grateful.

In the meantime, I saw the Pulmonary specialist, who decided in the end, that I had a pneumonitis, an inflammation of the lung, as a reaction to the Taxol. He told me it was actually quite small. He was convinced that I could continue with a Taxane as long as I was treated with steroids, which would hopefully protect me from any further allergic reactions. This was precisely what my friend had said he would do. When I met with my oncologist after three weeks, she told me she had decided to do just that, except she would use Taxotere and give it to me in smaller increments, but do it weekly. Apparently, that was what they were giving to patients with metastatic breast cancer. I could not believe my ears! Now I was going to get Taxotere, which was what I had wanted in the first place. I had a reaction to the Taxol, not bad enough to kill me, as it did most of the patients in the literature, but just enough to get me switched to the Taxotere. How wonderful was that! God does work in mysterious ways!

I was started on a weekly regimen of Taxotere which was even more dose densed, so it was not surprising that the side effects were pretty severe. Aside from all the other side effects that I was already familiar with, I developed neuropathy, which is a common side effect of the Taxanes. My hands and feet felt like they were on fire, and I had numbness and tingling in some parts of my body, while I had no feeling in some other parts of my body. I must be a glutton for punishment though, because in-spite of all these, I had some tricks up my sleeves to ensure that I got more than my share of the Taxotere. Since the dosage was measured by weight, I always wore my thickest sweaters and pants plus an extra camisole under my blouse (this was in the Fall, so I was able to do all that). I would also wear my heavy shoes which I did not take off when I was being weighed. All this, in an effort to get a little bit more of the Taxotere, as a way of making sure that the cancer cells were getting more of the drug. Actually, by the time I was down to the last 3 sessions of chemo, I asked Joan, my oncology nurse practitioner, if I could have 2 or 3 extra doses. I guess in my mind, I just wanted the insurance, that all the cancer cells would be bombed to oblivion! Her wise answer was to wait and see how I felt when I had completed the course of the chemotherapy. She was concerned that the neuropathy might become permanent, if I took too much of the drug. In the end, the side effects were so bad, especially the neuropathy, that I just felt relieved when I finally had my last session. Both Joan and I decided my body could not tolerate any more Taxotere.

The chemotherapy was followed by radiation. This was to ensure that any possible remaining cancer cells in the chest and neck area would be killed by the radiation. My main problem with it was the fatigue and local skin irritation. Otherwise, it was nowhere near as difficult as the chemotherapy. By the time I finished with the radiation, I was still suffering from remnants of the side effects of the chemotherapy, mainly the inability to enjoy food, because of damage to my taste buds. I remember, on the last day of my radiation treatment, I excitedly told my husband I wanted to celebrate. I had been craving for pizza for a long time! I was sick and tired of eating clam chowder, which had been my staple food during my many months of chemotherapy. I had difficulty with chewing and swallowing solids because of the sores in my tongue and mouth, hence I was limited to soups, and clam chowder was it for me. Well, I had no problems chewing the pizza at this point, but it still tasted like cardboard! I would have to wait for several more weeks, before I could enjoy eating again. At any rate, I was just very happy that the whole physical ordeal was over!

# Chapter 3

# The Guilt

During those difficult days of my chemotherapy and radiation, I was practically useless around the house. I was always feeling tired, and because of my neuropathy, I could not even help with any of the chores, such as cleaning up the kitchen, cooking, or doing the dishes. Touching cold water with my hands was agonizingly painful. I felt so sorry for my husband! Not only did he have to do everything around the house, he also had the job to keep the office going in my absence. He had to search high and low for a doctor to take care of my patients, while I was going through my treatment and unable to take care of them. I felt guilty watching him doing a thousand things, looking like the proverbial chicken with its head cut off. While I, on the other hand, did nothing but lie around and do a lot of thinking. I felt so guilty! I kept thinking I had brought all these problems upon myself because of my carelessness with my mammogram. And now my family was suffering as a consequence. I realized that I had put this emotional and physical burden on my husband and my children. My children had to take time off from their busy schedules to help us out.

My older daughter and her husband were in the midst of preparing to transfer their family from California to Germany, so needless to say they were very busy, but they took time off from their preparations to come to Michigan. While Trinnie accompanied me on my consultations with different oncologists and helped me to sort out the pros and cons of where to get my chemotherapy, her husband Michael, who is a lawyer, got busy with taking care of the business aspects of the practice. Both my sons also came home. The older one, Alberto Jr., with his wife Jade, came from Seattle and the younger one, George, with his then fiancee Maureen, now his wife, came from San Francisco, to spend time with us and give us emotional support. Veronica, our youngest child, came from New York to be with us, at a time when she should have been doing auditions. I was of course very grateful for their help, which was invaluable to us, but at the same time it made me feel very guilty.

The "if onlys" were killing me. If only I had kept close tabs on my yearly exam schedules, I would not have missed my mammograms; if only I had missed one year instead of two, the breast cancer would have been diagnosed in an early stage, and my situation would not have been so dire. Our family would not have had to go through this much turmoil. The thought that I could possibly die in a short span of time was something that I had to face. That was bad enough. But the thought that it would have been brought about by my own carelessness, compounded the guilt. I cried a lot whenever I was alone at home. The burden of guilt lay oppressively heavy on my shoulders. I was very careful however, not to let my husband know how I really felt. I did not want to burden him with more than what he was already going through. I figured since he is not medically oriented, he would think that as long as I was undergoing treatment, I would be fine. I thought that if I maintained a calm demeanor in his presence, he would think all was well. I didn't know then, that he had actually googled the statistics on breast cancer, and he knew exactly how grave the situation was. He actually knew what the percentage survival rate was in my stage of the disease. It was not very good! I would know about this, a few years later. So much for trying to keep medical secrets in this day and age of the Internet.

At any rate, it was very difficult keeping my thoughts to myself. All through my married life, my husband has been my confidant. I have never kept any secrets from him. He is the only one, with whom I could share anything and everything I have in my mind. That time however, I could not share my fears with him. He had too much to worry about already and I felt that unloading my burden of guilt and fears on him would be so unfair to him. I talked to Sue, the nurse-liaison at the Dept of Oncology at St Joe's about my emotional difficulties. She suggested that I see a psychiatrist who was versed in treating patients with cancer. I think she felt that he would be able to help me deal with my fears as well as my guilt feelings. She gave me the name and phone number of a psychiatrist she knew. I fully intended to avail myself of his services. However, I never got around to making the appointment. Something happened that made it unnecessary. Looking back now though, I think what I should have done, was to get involved in the support group meetings that Susan had suggested initially. At that time,

I could not see how sharing my feelings with others, or listening to other breast cancer patients share their thoughts about their illness would help me. Now however, if someone were to ask me, if I thought it would be a good idea, I would definitely say yes. I think being able to share information, as well as feelings would be helpful.

Anyway, there was one question that kept going through my mind during this period. The question was not why me? I am a woman, I have breasts, so of course I am a candidate for breast cancer. Even men, are not totally exempted from this disease. However, the question that kept going through my mind was, why did this happen to me? I kept saying to myself, "why did this happen to me? There has to be a reason for this." I felt that I had none of the predisposing factors for breast cancer. There was no family history, I had my first child before age 30, I breastfed all my children, and I had never been seriously overweight. Sure, I liked to eat red meat, but I knew other women who were more fond of their steaks than I was, and they did not have cancer. So if I did not have the aforementioned predispositions to breast cancer, why did this happen to me? This was the question that kept going over and over in my mind. I am a firm believer that things happen for a reason. So I kept telling myself that there had to be a reason for this to happen. There had to be a message here somewhere.

# Chapter 4

# The Message

One day, during one of my introspections, it dawned on me! I was born a Catholic, raised in a Catholic family, educated in Catholic institutions, so of course, I believed in God! But in all my 63 years, where was God in my life? He was a far-away God, up there in His heaven. Someone, I called on from time to time, to ask for favors for me, or for my family and again from time to time, to say thank you for favors granted. There had never been any question in my mind, that He was a very benevolent God. He certainly had given me more than I could have asked for, a doting husband, four great kids, and at the time of my diagnosis, three lovely granddaughters, and a large extended family. All of these were blessings, which I thoroughly enjoyed and for which I was very grateful. But I had been too busy enjoying the good life, He had given me, that I had forgotten to put Him at the center of my life, which is where He should always have been. He was not the focus of my life, which He should always have been. In short, in all that busyness, I had relegated Him to the periphery of my life. This was a new discovery for me! I had always thought of myself as a good Catholic. After all, I went to mass on Sundays and Holydays of Obligation without fail. In my mind, I was trying to follow the Ten Commandments as well as I could. My husband and I were relatively generous in our monetary contributions to the parish and other charitable organizations. I probably even thought of myself as a "better Catholic" than some people I knew. What a misguided thought! As I lay there, sort of reviewing my life, I realized how sadly lacking it had been in spirituality.

I thought of how I had always been such an avid reader since my high school days. I had read all kinds of novels, fictions and non-fictions. I could remember scouring the city libraries in Manila for books that I could not find in the school library. My favorite vacation, was the time I spent a whole month doing nothing from morning to late afternoon, but reading all kinds of books, without anybody bothering me. It happened when I went back to my hometown, for my vacation, the summer after premed. I went to our old house, which was now vacant, and found out there were so many books there. It was a treasure trove of all kinds of books, mystery stories, romance stories, even some classics. I had not known that my parents were such book lovers. At that time, I was staying at my grandparent's house in another part of town, so I made a deal with the maid. She would pack my lunch for the day, and as soon as breakfast was over, off I would go to the old house and she was not to tell anybody where I was, so my day would not be interrupted. I would just get back to my grandparent's house in time for dinner. It seems funny now to me, that at age 18, I thought that was the greatest way to spend my vacation days.

During the Tech bubble in the late 90's to early 2000, I got involved in the stock market. I was reading all the financial magazines and newspapers every day. I knew all the CEOs of the important tech companies that I was invested in. Sad to say, in all this time, I had never read the bible, or any other spiritual books. I had never read the life of any of the saints, and I had no interest in acquainting myself with them either. Except for the rosary, which I liked because I related it to the Blessed Mother, I was not familiar with some of the common Catholic devotions, such as the Divine Mercy devotion, which I found out later was a very popular one. While I was sick, I got a lot of prayer cards, medals, rosaries, and some devotional prayers, aside from the usual get well cards, from patients and friends. The Divine Mercy devotion was sent to me by the mother of my son's girlfriend at that time. I read the entire booklet from cover to cover, and later on, it became one of my favorite prayers.

My knowledge of the bible was limited to the bits and pieces I would hear from the gospel readings at masses, so I decided to start reading the bible. Since I could not do anything else, I had all the time in the world to do a lot of reading. I decided I would start with the life of Jesus, according to the four gospels. But the more I read, the more questions I had, such as why did Jesus say that or why did Jesus do that? I realized I needed someone to guide me through the bible, someone like a spiritual psychiatrist, I thought. I needed someone to answer all the questions that I had regarding the teachings and the actions of Jesus. So I called up Manresa, hoping to get a Jesuit priest as a spiritual guide. In the Philippines, the Jesuits were known as very good theologians. However, I was told that the priests were very busy, but that I could possibly instead join in the Ignatian Lay exercises. But when I got the enrolment form, I realized I was probably not ready for the exercises. From the questions they were asking, it seemed to me, they were expecting people who were more advanced in their spirituality than I was. So I was told to get some instructions from one of the lay people who had graduated from the Ignatian exercises. I was told anyone of them could probably help me in my desire to learn more about Jesus and help me to develop a better relationship with Him.

At about this time, my husband and I had gotten into the habit of going to the 7 am mass at the Monastery of the Blessed Sacrament. I will never forget that one morning, when I woke up around 5:30 as usual, but instead of getting dressed and ready to go to mass, I decided to forgo the mass that day. I was not feeling well, and it was a really chilly morning in late October or early November. But somehow, I kept looking at the clock on the headboard. Then at 6:35 I jumped out of bed and told Alberto we were going to mass. I don't know what made me change my mind! All I know was, suddenly, I felt an urgency to go to mass. The problem was, it would take us at least 15 minutes to get to the Monastery. We barely had 10 minutes to get ready. There was no time to shower, no time to put on my make-up. I only had time to wash my face, brush my teeth, grab a bandana to cover my bald head, put on a pair of pants and blouse and get out the door. Funny thing is, at any other time, under no circumstance, could you get me out of the house without make-up! And if I ever needed make-up so badly, this was the time! I had no hair, no eyebrows, no eyelashes, and my skin was blotchy and sallow from the effects of the chemotherapy. Somehow, that morning, as soon as I had decided to go to mass, I couldn't care less about the make-up or the lack of it.

We got to the Monastery just as the mass was starting. It started pretty much just like any other mass at the Monastery, beautiful and solemn, with the singing of the psalms. Then came the homily. The first reading that morning was taken from the book of Samuel. It was about the war between the Israelites and the Philistines. The Israelites were so tired of being defeated. They wanted to win this war so badly! They even brought the Ark of the Covenant to the battlefield. Well, the Israelites were defeated and defeated ignominiously. It was a major catastrophe! Less than a third of the Israelite army was left to go home. Even the Ark of the Covenant was taken by the Philistines as part of the spoils of war. But since there was much fewer of them, and they happened to have a good leader, the Israelites actually became a much better people. They went back to their covenant with God. Then, in conclusion of his homily, Father Martin said, sometimes in our lives, something happens that we think is a major catastrophe, but later when we look back, we realize it was actually a blessing, just as the defeat of the Israelites turned out to be a great blessing for them.

As he was saying these words, I was seating at the second row, thinking he is looking at me! It hit me! This was the message I had been looking for all along! This was telling me that the breast cancer was not the major catastrophe that I had thought it was. It was actually a blessing! God was saying something to me through it. He was telling me, it was time for a change in my priorities. I felt as if He was putting His stamp on me. He was calling me to a deeper, more personal relationship with Him. After the mass was over, I sat there for a while, thinking about what had just happened. Now I knew why things had happened the way they did! I realized that had I been diagnosed with very early cancer i.e. stage 0 or stage 1, it would not have made any change in my life, because I would have known that my chances for survival would be great, and there would not have been this strong need to cling to God. I had to experience the depths of total helplessness and hopelessness to bring me to God's door. I could feel the dark cloud of depression vanishing like mist in the morning sun. Most of all, the oppressive weight of the burden of guilt was lifted from my shoulders.

I walked out of the chapel that morning feeling very lighthearted. I never again cried because of the cancer, for now I knew, that there was a reason for my missing my mammograms and discovering the breast cancer at an advanced stage. This is not to say, that we should not try to do our yearly mammograms faithfully, so as to discover breast cancer as early as possible. We know that the only way to defeat breast cancer is to discover it as early as possible! Unfortunately in my case, I had completely been unaware, that so much time had elapsed between my mammograms. It was carelessness on my part, for which there is no excuse. However, that morning's homily and the homilist's conclusion was a much needed balm, not only to assuage a guilty conscience, but also to give me a spiritual perspective to an unfortunate situation. I look back now on that morning, as truly the beginning of my conversion journey. I knew then, that however short or long a life He would give me, I would want to spend it trying to forge a more loving personal relationship with Him. Strange as it may sound, since that morning, I have thought of the breast cancer as a gift. I went from despair and hopelessness, to a sense of gratitude to God, for opening my eyes in time. As devastating a diagnosis as cancer is, there is something to be grateful for, about it. With cancer, you do not die in a day, or a month, or maybe even years. It gives one the time to review one's life and make the necessary changes that can bring a fuller, richer, more joyful life, albeit a shorter one maybe.

Nowadays, when I hear of the sad news about someone being diagnosed with cancer, I am of two minds. There is no question that a diagnosis of cancer is an excruciatingly painful one for the patient and the family. I feel sadness and compassion. But there is this part of me, that says, this person is being given the time to change things in his or her life, that may need changing. I hope and pray, that person uses whatever time there is to make needed changes in his or her relationships, whether it be with family, friends or with God. It could be, that time is being given to heal wounded relationships. It maybe the time to say I love you, I'm sorry forgive me, or I forgive you. And being given that time is certainly something to be grateful for.

This brings to my mind the story of a young hairdresser I met recently He was the youngest of three siblings. Apparently, in high school, he realized that he was gay, and that he did not want to go to college as his two siblings did. Instead, he wanted to be a hairdresser. His father was very upset about this, and this produced a rift between them. I could feel the sadness in his voice when he talked about how differently his father treated him, from the way he treated his older siblings. His father hardly spoke to him, making life at home intolerable. He decided to move out and live on his own. He became quite successful in his career. The only thing missing in his life was the approval of his father. He wanted his father to be proud of him in the same way he was proud of his other children. He kept hoping that someday, the reconciliation with his father, that he longed for so much, would come about. His hope was that his father would mellow as he got older and eventually would learn to accept him for who he was. Unfortunately, his father died suddenly of a massive heart attack, putting an end to any hopes of reconciliation. I could not help thinking while he was recounting his story, that if his father had been diagnosed with cancer instead, there might have been time for either one of them, to make the first step towards repairing their broken relationship. They might have been given the time to forgive, to forget the anger, and to rebuild the love between them.

In my case, I am such a type A personality, that I always thought someday, hopefully when I was much older, I would just keel over suddenly and die of a massive heart attack. But now, I think that God in His great mercy and wisdom, decided to ignore my own death scenario. He knew some things needed changing in my life. Somewhere in my journey through life, the thought, that God should be first and foremost, had been forgotten. As I have said before, in all that busyness in my life, God had been taken out of the center and the focus of my life and relegated to the periphery. I now believe that the breast cancer was a wake-up call for me. For this, I will always be grateful to Him.

# Chapter 5

# The Sanctuary

As soon as I was able to drive by myself again, I made the habit of going to the Monastery of the Blessed Sacrament at 13 mile and Middlebelt, every afternoon for my holy hour. Since it was the only church that was open from morning till five in the afternoon, it became my sanctuary. Somehow, when I was there, I felt at peace and more hopeful. I loved the fact that the Blessed Sacrament was always exposed, and I would feel that Jesus was truly there, listening to everything I had to say. I would pray the Divine Mercy at exactly 3 o'clock. The pamphlet said that Jesus had said to St Faustina, that the greatest amount of mercy and love would flow from His Heart at that exact time, because that was the time of His greatest suffering on the cross. And whatever was asked of Him at that moment would not be refused, unless it was against His will. I asked Him for complete healing, physical and spiritual. I had long conversations with Him. I reminded Him that He had said, "ask and it shall be given, seek and you will find, knock and the door will be opened." This was something I had gleaned from my recent bible readings. I would say to Him, "here I am Lord, asking, seeking, knocking." I would also remind Him, that in my readings, I could find no instance in the bible, when He refused to heal anyone who asked. And there were times, when He healed them, even when they were not asking, as in the case of the blind paralytic man at the pool of Bethesda, and when He gave back the widow of Nain her son's life, because He felt compassion for her. Then just to make my appeal stronger, I would turn to the Blessed Mother for her intercession by praying the rosary, finishing it with the Memorare, one of my favorite petition prayers to the Blessed Mother. Then I would read the Psalms. I especially loved Psalm 91, which I would read over and over again. There was always that quivering feeling of fear inside me. I often wondered, if I would even make it through the chemotherapy. Somehow, reading this Psalm would calm me down. This Psalm promises that if you cling to God and make Him your refuge, He would protect you from all evils. He would have His angels hold you up and keep you from harm's way. I needed that reassurance so badly! But then, I also needed to prepare myself for the possibility that things would not turn out as well as I was hoping for, so I would then pray Psalm 23, The Lord is my Shepherd. This was my way of telling myself, that if I had to walk through the "dark valley of death," it would not be so bad, knowing that the Lord would walk with me through it.

There were times, when I would just sit there, watching the other people who came in, at the same time I did, and wondered what their problems might be. I did not know any of them personally, but in my mind, I felt a certain kinship with them. I knew we were all in some kind of trouble. Initially, there were three gentlemen, who were always at the chapel at the same time I was there. I could feel we were all praying very hard. Then two of them eventually stopped coming. I hoped that they had just moved from the area and hopefully were going to another church. But in my heart, I knew that was just wishful thinking. I particularly remember the one gentleman, who came every afternoon at about the same time that I did. I was pretty sure he had cancer. He kept getting thinner and thinner. The last time I saw him, he looked so gaunt and a little unkempt, as though he did not have the strength anymore, nor the desire to look good. I was saddened, but not surprised when I did not see him anymore after that day. All these occurrences were very unsettling to me.

The fear that something would go wrong imminently was always with me. Seeing the others drop out, one by one, made my fears even more real to me. At times, after my prayers, I would just sit there and take a little nap. It was the only time in my entire day when I felt some semblance of peace. Although I tried not to show it, for most of the day I felt bruised and battered inside. I was a bundle of frayed nerves. The Monastery of the Blessed Sacrament became for me, my oasis in a desert of fear. The problem was, being a physician, I was aware of all the possibilities. I knew all the statistics. That was not very good for my psyche.

Looking back now, the only thing that kept me going was my faith in the Blessed Mother's willingness and ability to intercede for me. Yes, the odds were definitely not good, but she had always come through for me in the past. I knew she was my most powerful ally in my battle against the cancer! In my opinion, whether one calls it, positive thinking, or faith, it certainly was an important factor in my healing: physically, emotionally, and spiritually. In any case, the Monastery of the Blessed Sacrament became a place of refuge for me. For that, I have always been very grateful to the Cloistered Dominican nuns for keeping the chapel open the whole day, giving people like me and many others a sanctuary.

# Chapter 6

# The Awakening

This was also about the time, as I have said, that I had decided to avail myself of the services of the lay instructor at Manresa. During one of the sessions I had at Manresa, my instructor asked me what I was doing with my time. When I told her about the things I was doing, the holy hour, going to daily mass etc, she looked at me for a while, then said, "Lourdes, are you trying to earn God's love?" I thought about it for a few minutes, and said yes, I guess so. She then said to me, "there is nothing you can do to earn His love, it is freely given, nothing that you do or don't do can change His love for you." Nobody had ever told me that! When I was growing up, the God that I learned about was more of a just God than a loving God. He was a God to be feared! You better made sure that you did not end up in the wrong side of His list. He would reward the good and punish the bad, period. You either went to heaven or to hell based on your merits. As a child growing up in a fairly religious community, the concept of our relationship with God was very simplistic. The idea was, God was this very powerful Being up in Heaven, watching our every move. If you were good, then He would reward you and you would end up in Heaven. If on the other hand, you were naughty or just not behaving according to His rules, you would burn forever in Hell. That was a very scary thought! I think this made for very obedient and well behaved children. But I think, even the adults in the community also believed this to be true.

When I look back, I realize that in our religion classes, we learned mostly about the God of the Old Testament. We learned mostly about the stories of God punishing the Israelites for their misbehaviors. There was no talk about a very merciful and loving God, Who is constantly giving us grace, so He can strengthen us in our weaknesses, and bring us to heaven, because that is where He actually wants all of us to be. Hearing the Manresa instructor say that God's love was freely given, even when it was not deserved, showed me a very different picture of God. That was welcome news for me, because if truth be told, I had always felt a little alienated from God. I felt rather uncertain about my relationship with Him. He was Someone, I obeyed out of fear, not out of love. I think it is very difficult, to really love someone that you fear! My picture of God was that of the Old Testament God, who was always getting angry with the Israelites and punishing them or threatening to punish them. This was probably the reason, why I had always felt the need to cling to the Blessed Mother, as a child would cling to its mother, thinking she was the softer side of heaven, and she would smooth things out for me. Thankfully, as I started reading the bible more, especially parts of the Old Testament, the picture of God's relationship with His chosen people, became a little clearer to me. Yes, He got angry with them a lot of times, but they were deserving of His anger! They were often turning their backs on Him, completely forgetting all that He had done for them. Many times, they turned away from their covenant with Him. But in-spite of all that, He never gave up on them! He never said, "I have had enough of your intransigence!" He kept taking them back over and over again, pretty much the way a loving parent does, with a wayward child. But this knowledge all came later.

That day, as I was driving home from Manresa, I kept thinking about what my instructor had said, that God's love was freely given, that we did not need to do anything to get it. So then why should I be doing all that I was doing, if it was not needed? Wasn't it all just a waste of my time? Then, I got to thinking about my parents. I never had any doubt that they loved me very much. We were not a huggy, kissy family, we were not the type to say I love you at the end of conversations. My parents were the typical Filipino parents, very strict, but nevertheless, I knew I was loved. I knew that their love for me was there, no matter what. So how did I react to that? I toed the line! Whatever my parents told me to do, I did. Whatever they told me not to do, I did not do, no arguments. I just wanted to please them as much as I could. It was my way of saying to them, "I love you too, very much." So my thoughts then turned to this new revelation, that God loved me unconditionally, pretty much like my parents did. I knew now, that there was nothing I needed to do, for Him to love me, but I decided

I would continue to do what I had been doing. This would be my way of saying to Him, Who loves me so much, "I love you too, very much." It felt good to know, that finally, my relationship with Him would be one of love not of fear. The more I thought about this new-found relationship I had with God, I knew there were other things I needed to do. This was just the beginning of the journey.

# Chapter 7

# God's Whispers

It was uncanny, but about a year or a year and a half before I got my diagnosis, sometimes when I was driving to work, a thought would just pop into my head, "what are you doing with your life?" I knew what the question was about. I thought that I was feeling a little guilty, because I had been with my parish for more than twenty years but I had not been involved in any parish activity. It was easy to write a check when they asked for some donations, but giving of my time or my efforts was another thing altogether. I kept thinking I wanted to teach catechism. I also wanted to be a Eucharistic minister for the sick. Yet every time there was a notice in the parish bulletin, asking for volunteers for these activities, I chose to ignore them. My excuse always, was that, I was too busy at that time, and I would just wait till I retired, to get involved. I did not want anything impinging on my "busy life." But the truth was, I was enjoying my practice very much and the perks that went with it, that I had no intentions of retiring until I just could not do it anymore mentally or physically. I figured, it would take a very long time. The odd thing was, on more than a couple of occasions, when I would make the excuse "not now", "when I retire", I distinctly remember a thought coming to my mind saying "what if there is no time?" I chose to ignore that too. I even remember a recurring thought that would come to my mind in those times. I would compare myself to a ship. I knew where the port was. But instead of heading straight for it, I opted to meander, to enjoy the distractions along the way. I even had the audacity, to say to myself, that it was God, who was giving me all the resources to enjoy the distractions. Aside from the fact, that I was busy raising a family and managing a busy medical practice, I was just positively enjoying life, parties with friends, vacations in faraway places with the family, and working hard, to make sure we were financially secure and able to afford the good life. Those were the things that were uppermost in my mind. I guess, as many younger people do, I figured the time for seriously seeking a deeper, personal relationship with God would come later, when it was more "convenient" for me. Looking back now, I see that my focus was a little askew. It was as though, I said to God, as some busy young people subconsciously do, "Lord, just wait there, right now I don't have much time for You. Someday, when my plate is not too full, I will come back and pay more attention to You." That attitude probably stems from the idea that God will always patiently wait and will always be there. At any rate, that was probably my intention, not thinking that God might get impatient and take things into His own hands.

There was something else that was going on in my life at that time, that looking back now, I think may have had a bearing on the subsequent events that occurred in my life, a year and a half later. I remember on Wednesdays, which was my day off, the drug agents would invite me to play golf with them, because apparently, that was what a lot of the male physicians did on their day off. They would laugh, when I would say, sorry I can't, that is my day for mopping my kitchen floor. And indeed that was what I did on my day off, mop the kitchen and bathroom floors. While I mopped the floor, I would sing a song that I had learned from my time with a group called BLD (Bukas Loob sa Dios). In English, it means open yourself to God. It was just one of those short songs that had a catchy tune. I don't know why I chose to sing that particular song, except it was a very easy song to sing. It went like this:

> Change my heart oh God, make it ever true.
> Change my heart oh God, make me be like you.
> You are the Potter, I am the clay.
> Mold me and change me, this is what I pray,
> Change my heart oh God, make it ever true.
> Change my heart oh God, make me be like You.

I would sing it over and over again until I finished mopping. Now when I look back, I think maybe God was listening and decided to take me up on it! Maybe, just maybe, He was getting a little impatient with me at this time. There is a saying, God talks to us in whispers, but if we don't listen, then He might just knock us over the head. I think that was exactly what He did. Since I was not listening to His whispers, He decided to hit me on the head, and in the process turned my life upside down. I like to think that God, in His great mercy, decided to wake me up from my apathy. It has been almost 7 years now since my diagnosis, and when I go over in my mind, the things that have happened, the changes in my life since then, I can only say "thank you Lord, for your Divine Providence, for "the moments rightly placed" in my life, that changed its course so drastically, but in my opinion so beautifully." This journey has been so spiritually fulfilling for me, that for as long as I live, I will always feel very grateful to God. As I have said before, there have been so many changes in my life since my illness, changes that have enriched my life and have brought me so much joy. I now teach catechism at my parish, and I do Eucharistic ministry once a week to the patients at St Joes. I find both of these activities very rewarding, emotionally and spiritually. I have also become more involved with my parish and I have developed friendships with many of my co-parishioners who come to daily mass. All of these have added so much happiness and balance to my life. Sometimes I think, why did it take so long for me to discover all this? Why couldn't I have been led to this life much earlier so I could have had a long time to enjoy it? I guess, as another song that I learned from BLD says, "everything happens in God's time." Maybe, if the breast cancer had occurred much earlier in my life, my reactions might have been different, and I might not have been ready to respond to God's grace. Maybe, we should just accept grace when it comes and be grateful for it.

# Chapter 8

# The Mass

When I consider in my mind, what has been the most tangible change in my spiritual life, since I began this conversion journey, without doubt, it is the way I feel about the mass. As I have said before, I was born a Catholic and raised in a Catholic family, so of course like most Catholics, I went to mass on Sundays and Holydays of obligation. And that was the operative word-obligation! Mass was just something I needed to do as part of my religion. It was one of those things, that as a Catholic, I was obliged to do. There was no joy in it for me. When I think back now, I realize that this unfortunate attitude could have been the result of my childhood observations. Ironically, I grew up in a small town in the Philippines, that by most metrics, seemed very religious, as most small towns in my country seem to be. I remember the frequent processions all over town, celebrating the feast days of the saints or the Blessed Mother. We would track all over town, reciting the rosary or the novena for a specific saint. Most of the time, at the end of the procession, we would end up in somebody's house for dinner or snacks. Of course, as kids we enjoyed this very much. The month of May was always a fun month for us kids. It was the month dedicated to the Blessed Virgin Mary and every afternoon the young girls called the Virgines, would dress up in white gala dresses with our hair adorned with beautiful crowns of flowers. We would participate in a ceremony giving tribute to the Blessed Virgin, by offering prayers, songs and fresh flowers for her altar. As usual it would end up in snacks for the kids.

On Sundays, the church would be filled to capacity and you could tell from the way the women dressed whose devotees they were. They would be dressed in green for St Joseph, brown for St Anthony and white dress with blue sash for the Lady of Lourdes, or just plain blue for the Immaculate Conception. Sundays were always very festive, and it seemed like most of the townspeople showed up for mass. Unfortunately however, there seemed to be the prevailing idea that the first part of the mass, which we call the Liturgy of the Word, was not important. A lot of people would come to mass after the homily (called the sermon then). The idea was, as long as you were in time for the offertory, which was the beginning of the second part of the mass, then you had fulfilled your "obligation." Worse yet, there was a practice of a lot of the men to go out of the church to smoke, or talk among themselves, while the gospel was being read and they would come back in, after the sermon was over. This lent to the idea that the first half of the mass was not at all important. I also remember, that a lot of the old ladies were praying their rosaries during the mass. I love the rosary, but as beautiful a prayer as it is, I don't think it has a place in the mass. We should pray the rosary before the mass, as we do at St Owens, or after the mass, a practice in some other churches I have attended, but definitely not during the mass. When I look back now, I think that unfortunately, those old ladies in my hometown just did not understand what the mass was truly all about. They probably had no idea of the significance and the true beauty of the Holy Sacrifice of the Mass.

Growing up in that atmosphere, I'm not surprised that my concept of the mass was quite flawed. As an adult, I was habitually late for mass. I did not pay much attention to the homily, and worse yet, on many occasions, I would sit there critiquing it. If I didn't think that the homilist was doing a "good job" I would say to myself, "I would develop this topic differently," so instead of listening, I would be off on a tangent, doing my own "theme". Oh what arrogance! At the same time, I had no idea then, about transubstantiation, that as Catholics we believe in. In all the years of my going to mass and receiving communion, I had never been made aware of the Real Presence of Jesus at communion. I always thought of the bread and wine as just symbols, to remind us of what Jesus had done at the last supper. So how could I have known then, what a great privilege the mass is, and what an awesome gift the Holy Eucharist is!

It is odd, how a confluence of events led me to appreciate the mass for what it truly is. It started with a question I had, when I first started reading the bible. I would think, now why did Jesus do what he did at the last supper? Why did He decide to institute the Holy Eucharist, instead of just saying to the apostles, "I have been with you for the past 3 years, I have taught you everything I want you to know; tomorrow they are going to kill me. I want you all to live as I have taught you and to preach the gospel to the entire world." But no, He made a point of instituting the Holy Eucharist. At this point in my life, through my association with the BLD group, I was already aware of the concept of transubstantiation,(that the bread and wine at the moment of consecration are changed completely into the body and blood of Jesus).The more I thought of it, the more I came to the conclusion that this was proof that Jesus loved us so much, He did not want to leave us! I especially felt that this privilege of being in His Real Presence, was such a special gift to those of us who were born after His death. The apostles and the other disciples were fine. They had had the privilege of enjoying His company, sharing meals with him, and having conversations with Him. But for those believers who were born after His death, the communion is the only way that we can experience being in His Physical Presence too. That thought gave me a sense of His great love for me. It made me very happy, to think, that He cared so much for me, that He wanted to be with me, not just in an abstract concept, but truly united with Him physically. I know why this mattered so much to me. Somewhere in this book, I express how in the past, I had always felt "unlovable" to Jesus. It was not a very good feeling!

This was also the time, when I was trying to read Revelation. Well, I couldn't read it. After a few pages I put it down. It was too gory for me. I decided to talk to my son George, about my reaction to Revelation. I knew he had taken bible studies and was into apologetics. I knew he had a strong faith and I had always admired him for that. I figured he would be the one to help me understand the complexities of Revelation. He asked me if I had read the Lamb's Supper, a book by Scott Hahn, which was one of three books he had sent me when I was sick. I had not. He told me to read it because the author talks about Revelation in that book. As soon as we finished our conversation, I decided to read the book. It's funny, but I don't remember now, what Scott Hahn said about Revelation, but I remember what he said about the mass. Many of us have had the experience of being in a truly breathtakingly beautiful place, causing us to say, "This is heaven on earth," or experiencing such joy and contentment as to say, "This is heaven." Well, in his book Scott Hahn talks about the mass, as the actual "heaven on earth". He talks about The Real Presence of Jesus at the mass. This started me thinking, if I believe, that the mass is truly heaven on earth, why am I not trying to be there every opportunity I can get? And if the bread is the Real Presence, why am I not availing myself of it every time I can? And why was I waiting for Sundays to avail myself of this great privilege, when He was there in the tabernacle, waiting for me every day? I thought of the amount of money we spend and the efforts we take, to see some celebrity in a concert, and yet, Jesus is waiting for us at the mass every day, for free, and we say no, I will just see You on Sunday. I thought this behavior did not make sense. This was when I decided I would go to mass and receive communion everyday or at least as often as I can. I now believe that the mass is the greatest celebration of His love for us.

Just about the same time, that I was doing a lot of thinking about the mass, I attended a talk at the Shrine of the Little Flower church at Oak Park, by a Mexican lady, who claimed she had visions of the Blessed Mother. Somebody had given me a flyer about the event while I was at the Blessed Sacrament, so I convinced my husband that we should stop by, for a very short while, on our way to dinner at my sister's house. On any given day, when I get home from work, I usually do not have the energy or the desire to go out and attend "talks". As luck would have it however, my sister Alice was having a dinner for the whole family that night (it seems to me this was another one of those moments rightly placed, that I talk about in another part of this book).My husband and I decided we could stop by for a short while, since it was on the way to my sister's house anyway. I knew Alice would not mind if we were a little bit late, especially if I were to tell her what it was all about. When we came in, the church was completely packed, it was standing room only. It was odd, that the short time we were there, she was talking about the mass. Apparently, she was also one who did not pay much attention to the mass. She was always late for mass. The Blessed Mother chided her for her lack of the proper attitude towards the mass, and decided to show her what really happens at mass. She was given the privilege of seeing exactly what occurs during the mass. She said at mass every person has an angel standing by his or her side. She also saw that many saints were present at the mass. Then she described how at the moment of consecration, Jesus comes down to the altar and all the angels, the saints, and the Blessed mother kneel down with us in worship. I found it uncanny! This was the second time in a couple of weeks that I was made aware of the "heaven on earth" aspect of the mass. I loved the thought! Obviously, this has made attending mass very important for me.

Now I try to be at mass every day. I am never late for mass anymore. I try to be at least ten minutes early so as to have time to prepare myself for the mass, sort of center myself, get myself totally focused. I also take this time to thank God for the grace of being at church. I know that it is His grace that gets me to mass, especially on certain days when I am not feeling so inclined, to leave the comfort of my bed, early on a weekday morning. It is the promise of joy in the mass that gets me going. I can also honestly say now, that during the homily I am all ears! I have listened to homilies given by young priests, old priests, nuns and lay people. I have listened to erudite explanations of the gospels and some very simple ones and I have learned from them all. I remember when our parish priest was sick, a young priest from Nigeria was substituting for him. It was very difficult to understand him because of his accent. In previous times, I would probably just have decided to let my mind wander instead of trying to listen to him intently and understand what he was trying to convey. At the end of his homily, the take-home message was, that God does not just look at the results of the actions or decisions that we take in our life, but also at the efforts. I thought that was a very worthwhile and practical message, because how often do we resolve to follow God's will and fail. Heaven knows how many times, I have started the day with the best of intentions and by nighttime, when I review the events of my day, I find many instances where my best efforts were not good enough in bringing about the best results. It is very encouraging to know, that even our failed efforts are important in God's eyes. That morning, I was very glad that I made the effort to listen and understand the young priest's message. But the part of the mass that affects me most is the Liturgy of the Eucharist. I love the thought, that at the moment of consecration, the mass is truly "heaven on earth." At that moment, I close my eyes, and in my mind's eye I can see the picture that the Mexican lady described; Jesus at the altar, the Blessed Mother, the angels and saints worshipping at church with us. What a beautiful scene! Where else could I possibly want to be? Then of course the communion follows, and I am now given the awesome privilege of receiving the Lord. Sometimes, the joy and the gratitude can get so overwhelming, I cannot stop the tears from flowing.

# Chapter 9

# Spiritual readings

This conversion journey would not be complete without the help of spiritual books. They have played such an important role in my spiritual development. My love for reading has found a new venue. I now have a library of spiritual books in my bedroom. Aside from medical literature these are mostly the books I read now. I have learned so much from these books! I just wish I had been introduced to this genre a long time ago. So much to learn! For instance, the idea about "the fear of God." In the Old Testament and even in the Psalms they seem to tell us to fear God. I had that picture of a fearsome God in my mind since that was what I learned growing up. It was only after reading St. Teresa of Avila's autobiography that I learned what the "fear of God" should really mean. She says it should really be a fear of offending Him. Doesn't that make more sense? Why would you be so afraid of Someone who loves you very much and wants nothing but the best for you? That is actually the same question that another theologian, Fr. Antony F. Campbell, a Jesuit priest, seems to be asking in his book, God First Loved Us. St Therese of Lisieux said pretty much the same thing, when she said to her sister, mother Agnes, "Oh my dear mother, after so many graces, can I not sing with the Psalmist: How good is the Lord, His mercy endures forever! It seems to me that if all creatures had received the same graces I received, God would be feared by no one but would be loved to the point of folly; and through love, not through fear, no one would ever consent to cause Him any pain . . . . What a sweet joy it is to think that God is Just, that He takes into account our fragile nature. What should I fear then?" It certainly makes more sense to me, to be careful not to offend a God who is so loving and merciful than to be afraid of Him. I can actually relate to that, because as I have said before, the knowledge that my parents loved me so much, made me want to do everything that they wanted me to do, not because of fear but because of a desire to show them how much I loved them too and to try to please them in every way I could. Now the image of God that I have is so different from the image I had when I was growing up. In a similar manner, there is a book by the well-known Dutch spiritual writer, Henri Nouwen, entitled The Return of The Prodigal Son. It is one of the most interesting spiritual books I have read. I'm sure most Christians are familiar with the story because it is taken from one of Jesus' parables. But in the prologue he talks about the painting of Rembrandt portraying the homecoming of the prodigal son. He talks about the way Rembrandt painted the hands of the father, who of course represents God. One hand has a definitely masculine look while the other hand looks feminine with longer slender fingers. He explains it, as saying, that God loves us with the strong love of a father and the tender love of a mother. If I had never read the book, I know, I would never have noticed that feature, if I saw it a hundred times. Now when I go to Manresa, it gives me pleasure to stop by the picture which hangs on the corridor wall, to look at the hands and think of how God loves us.

Even as an adult, up to the time of my illness, I still had some issues with my relationship with Jesus. Actually, this was one of the reasons why I had wanted to have a spiritual guide. I think I needed someone to reassure me that Jesus loved me too. The thing is, who were the people that Jesus loved and surrounded Himself with? The apostles, a group of uneducated fishermen. And who were the people that Jesus seemed to dislike a lot? The Pharisees, a group of highly educated, arrogant, materially well-off people. Then I would think, in temperament, in education and in economic and social circumstances, I was more like the Pharisees than the apostles. That was a worrisome thought for me. I did not seem to fit in with Jesus' inner circle of friends! But then I started reading the book, Christianity Before Jesus. In it, the author talks about the different Jewish communities during the time of Jesus. He also talks about the frustration of Jesus with the Pharisees. They were the leaders of the society; they were the ones who were knowledgeable of the laws. They were supposed to help the poor and ignorant people follow the laws, but instead they made things more difficult for these people. He used the example of the prostitutes. If they wanted to ask for forgiveness from God and change their way of living, they needed to go to the temple and make sacrifices. This meant they would have to buy a sacrificial offering, as was the practice in those days. The problem was, the Pharisees deemed their money unacceptable because it came from sinful means. So how could they get out of their situation? In Jesus eyes the Pharisees, instead of lending a hand to those poor, sinful people to help them make their lives better, were actually making things more difficult for them. My conclusion was, aside from their resistance to accept Jesus' ministry, Jesus was angered by their lack of concern for the poor and the so-called sinners, who were trying to better themselves. It seems, the Pharisees were big on self-aggrandizement and short on concern for others. Jesus was justifiably angry with them not because of their high standards of living and education but because they were totally lacking in charity and humility. Jesus was simply telling the Pharisees not to be so arrogant and self-centered. Instead he wanted them to go out of their way to make things easier for those who were less fortunate than they were. Apparently, all that Jesus asks from all of us is to follow his example, by showing concern for the poor, the sick and whoever is in need of our help. That was good to know!

This is why every year in my catechism class I have decided to read with my class, Matt 25, 31-48. My 4th grade class consists of young boys and girls who come from relatively affluent families and I have no doubt that many of them will become successful professionals or business men or women in the future. I want them to be familiar with this gospel of St Matthew where Jesus talks about the end times. The idea that I want these kids to remember is that, in the end, the question we will be asked, is not how big a house we had, how much money we had in the bank, how profitable were our investments, or how much power we wielded while we lived. The question is simply, "What did you do for the least of my people?" This is not meant to discourage the kids from aspiring to be successful and prosperous in the future. After all, it is easier for someone who is successful and prosperous to be of help to others who are in need. Besides all our talents come from God and I am sure He would want all of us to develop our talents to the fullest and not waste His gifts to us. It is important however, I think, to acknowledge that all the good things we have are just gifts from Him and we are bound by the law of love to share those with the less fortunate.

There are so many other interesting books in my library now. It seems that one book leads to another, there are always more books to read. Without question, books not only inform but they can also help shape our way of thinking. I remember a friend of mine saying once, "We are only human beings, we are not saints." I can't remember the exact topic we were talking about, but it had something to do with how we were supposed to behave in a particular situation. Her idea was, we could not be expected to always do the right thing. That type of behavior would be expected of the saints, but not of ordinary human beings like us. I guess we all agreed with her at that time since nobody said anything to contradict her. But there is a book by Father Rolheiser entitled The Holy Longing, which I have read since, which says that we are all born with a certain dis-ease. That is, we are not completely at peace until that dis-ease is quelled. The premise, I think, is that there is a holy longing in each one of us that can find its complete satisfaction only in God. St Augustine pretty much said the same thing, when he said "You made us for yourself, Lord, and our hearts are restless until they rest in You." Father Rolheiser quotes Kierkegaard, in this book as saying, saints can will the one thing. Fr. Rolheiser contrasts that with how ordinary people like us are unable to do that, because somehow we cannot quite give up all the other pleasures of life. We want to love and serve God, but we also want to enjoy the material pleasures this world offers and therein lies the difference between the saints and the ordinary people like us. The example he gave was Mother Teresa, who willed to serve God and the poor, and that was what she did with her whole life, and what an amazing life that was! For that matter, you could site St Francis, who I think is one of the greatest saints, who gave up a life of wealth and prestige for the love of God. On the other hand, he gave the example of Princess Diana as someone like us, ordinary people. She was a good person, she did a lot of good things, but she could not quite give up the distractions of the good life. But now I say, if we all have that holy longing that will not be satisfied until we go to God, then we are all called to be saints. Forget St Francis, St Dominic, Mother Teresa, and all the other venerated saints. They are a totally different breed. Most of us can never even hope to be in their vicinity.

But I believe that ordinary people like us are called to be saints too. Not to become the venerated saints, but just ordinary everyday saints. I now believe that this journey we call life, is a journey to sainthood for everyone, and I like to think that along the way, a very merciful God gives us a lot of graces to get us to the goal. It may not be very evident in most of our lives, but I like to think we all progress at our own pace. I think in some lives the workings of grace may not be as obvious as in others, but it is there nevertheless. In some however, it shines through their daily lives, serving as examples for others. Such was the case of a friend of mine named Ely. We were neighbors but I didn't really get to know her well, until about 4 years before she died. She was a very prayerful person. Even at the worst time of her illness, when she became aware that the cancer had metastasized to her lungs, she was always concerned about praying for others who had health problems themselves. She was always at the daily mass at St Owens, where she was very much loved and respected because she always had time for anyone who needed advise, whether medical or personal in nature. She had a very strong faith. Even at the time she was suffering from Pancreatic cancer, her mantra was always "God is Great." Throughout her illness, she seemed to be always in sync with God's will. I admired her very much for that. She never questioned His mercy or His love even in times of great difficulty. Her faith in His Goodness seemed unshakeable. She was also a very generous person, with her time, with her resources, and with her skills. She was a retired physician, so she donated her time to give free consultations in a Downtown clinic for the poor. She only stopped doing that when she was already sick. When some people in the Filipino community needed help, she was there for them. During her wake, so many people came up to talk about specific instances of her kindness to them. It seemed like everyone who had known her, knew of instances when she opened her heart, her house or her wallet, to someone in need. She was a very kind, very compassionate person. I believe she was one person who truly lived the beatitudes. In my book, she was a true everyday ordinary saint. I am sure there are many like her out there, living lives of goodness, joyfully accepting God's will and bringing His love to others. These are the everyday ordinary people who are living lives of quiet sainthood. I can only pray, that this conversion journey will someday bring me to within a stone's throw to this kind of relationship with God and others. That is the goal.

# Chapter 10

# Moments Rightly Placed

One of the most interesting books I now have in my library is one that talks about "moments rightly placed." These are incidents in our lives that we might think of as happy coincidences or we could think of them as the unseen hand of God guiding us at certain moments of our lives. During my illness, and since then, I have experienced quite a few of those. When I was being prepared for surgery, the nurse and I were talking about cancer of the breast. She apparently had surgery herself for breast cancer 2 years before. I guess my surgeon had picked her to do my prep so she could give me encouragement. When the nurse left to see another patient, the lady in the next cubicle came up to me. She was there that day because her husband was going to have arthroscopic surgery. Anyway, she had heard us talking about breast cancer. She told me she had breast cancer 8 years ago. It was diagnosed late because the mass was behind the nipple and had been missed by the mammograms. She told me she had a total of 18 positive lymph nodes. She told me of her surgery and her chemotherapy and radiation. She had some tough times during the chemotherapy and the radiation, but there she was now, some eight years later, nicely coiffed and looking quite beautiful. As I was being wheeled out to surgery, she walked with me a short distance into the corridor, wished me luck, then went back to her husband's cubicle. When I woke up from the anesthetic, my surgeon came in and told me I had 17 positive lymph nodes! As I have said before that was devastating news, but when he said it, the first thought that came to my mind was, "she had 18 positive lymph nodes" and the picture in my mind was of her, looking beautiful and healthy, after 8 years. I didn't think of it then, but many months later, I would realize how providential it was that she was there that day. Was it just a happy coincidence that her husband was having arthroscopic surgery at the same hospital, on the same morning, I was having my surgery or was it God's way of saying to me, don't worry, here she is, she had one more lymph node than you and she is fine 8 years later. For me that was definitely a "moment rightly placed."

The incident with the Taxol, was certainly, in my mind, another evidence of the hand of God gently guiding me through the throes of chemotherapy. It also reminds me of what a priest once said to me. I had been telling him, that I had this problem of being unable to totally bend my will to God's will. I told him that most of the time, I would say to God, please let me follow the example of Jesus in the garden, when He said, "not My will but Yours be done," but with the next breath, I would say, but if it is not against Your will, could You do it this way? I read a book once that said "let God be God, stop trying to micromanage Him." I guess that was what I was doing, trying to manage God. It was worrisome to me that I was always trying to bend God's will to mine instead of mine to His. I told the priest that my problem is, I am such a "control freak." I have this need to control all the events of my life. He said quite patiently to me, "no Lourdes, our problem as human beings is that we do not see the total picture, only God sees the total picture." He said, next time, just say, "Lord, I know your plans for me are better than my plans." In the case of my reaction to the Taxol, it was only later that I would look back and realize He made me react in such a way that it did not kill me, as it did many of the patients I had read about, but just enough to get me switched to taxotere, which was my drug of choice. It was only after His whole plan became clear to me, that I was able to say, "thank you Lord. You are wonderful!"

Another amazing example of moments rightly placed in my life happened about four years after my chemotherapy. In 2007, my husband and I joined a pilgrimage from Manresa to holy sites in France. While we were washing our faces and drinking from the faucets that line a part of the grounds at Lourdes, we met a Filipino nun, who was doing the same thing. We got into a conversation with her. She told us she was a sister of the Community of the Daughters of Charity, of which St Catherine Labourre of the Miraculous medal had been a member. She said that the uncorrupted body of St Catherine was in their chapel in Paris and she invited us to come visit her if we were ever in Paris. I was very interested because during my illness, a friend had sent me the miraculous medal and of course at that time I had no idea what it was all about. I knew we were going to be in Paris, but I wasn't sure if we would have time for the visit, so I did not pay much attention to the directions she was giving us. Well, the last day of our pilgrimage was in Paris. We spent the whole morning in a sightseeing tour of the city, culminating in a guided tour of the Notre Dame Cathedral. Then we were told the afternoon was free and we would be left to our own devices. Most of the people in the group decided to go shopping at The Lafayette store. We went along, but then, my husband and I were not too keen on shopping, so instead we went up to the floor where they had the restaurants since it was lunchtime. We were in the heart of Paris, we had the choice of many different cuisines and what did we eat? Chinese food! I guess old habits are just hard to break. At lunch, we remembered the nun's invitation and we thought how lucky that we had the whole afternoon free. We went back to the hotel to see if the desk clerk could direct us to the place but she only had a vague idea as to which part of the city it was located.

Anyway, we took the subway, which was just a walking distance from the hotel. My husband figured out which stop would be closest to our destination. After a short walk, we found ourselves in front of the chapel or so we thought. It was beginning to rain, so we hurried inside. The chapel was empty except for another couple, who were just getting ready to leave and at the very back of the chapel, sitting on a bench was an old woman. The chapel was rather bare. I can't remember now what the main altar had, but I couldn't see any evidence of any coffin where the body of the saint would be. When I looked around, I saw on the side a ramp going down so I decided to explore that, but there was nothing down there either. I went back up, and stood in front of a side altar that had a painting of the Blessed Virgin Mary. I prayed one Hail Mary and thought we might as well go back to the hotel. Anyway, it wasn't a very good day for touring on foot because of the rain. All of a sudden, I saw the old woman get up from the bench and walk towards me. She asked me in French if I was looking for the Miraculous medal and when I nodded, she proceeded to give me directions. From what I could understand, she was saying that the chapel was about a block or so away, and she gave me the name of the street and the number. I could not believe it! The French people are not exactly known for being overly helpful with foreigners, and in this case I didn't even ask for her help. I thanked her and told my husband the good news. When we got out of the chapel, the rain had stopped, so we decided to give it a try.

We found the chapel as she had directed. This one was filled with people and there at the sanctuary was a huge image of the Blessed mother of the Miraculous medal. Now I knew we were in the right place! As soon as I entered the chapel, my eye was directed to the left side of the sanctuary where I saw the body of a woman in a nun's habit lying in repose. I could not tell if it was an uncorrupted body or a wax reproduction but it certainly looked the same as the uncorrupted body of St Bernadette that we had seen several days before in Nevers. We knelt down to pray in front of this image, then Alberto took pictures and we decided to leave. As we left the chapel, I noticed on the side, a small opening which seemed to be a door of a small shop. We went in to buy some medals for family and friends. Almost at the same time that we walked in, the nun that we had met in Lourdes came in. It was her turn to be at the store. Apparently, the nuns took turns in being at the store. What were the odds that we would happen to be there at exactly the same time? Fortunately, from talking to her, I found out that the nun I had thought was St Catherine was actually the co-founder of the order. St Catherine was in the opposite side of the sanctuary and I had not even looked at that side. She also told us how we could get to St Vincent's chapel which was not too far from there. So after buying the medals and a small pamphlet about the life of St Catherine, we went back inside the chapel to see St Catherine. We said our prayers, took pictures of the uncorrupted body of St Catherine and just as we were getting ready to leave, the priest came out and started to celebrate the mass and of course we stayed for that. I couldn't help thinking, what a blessing it was, that we were at the chapel in time for the celebration of the mass, especially since our group had not had time for mass that morning.

After we had seen the chapel of St Vincent and we were on our way back to the hotel, Alberto and I marvelled at how things just seemed to have fallen in the right order starting with our "getting lost" in the other chapel, so we could meet up with the nun, get all the right information from her, and be in time for the mass at the Miraculous medal chapel. All in all, it was an extraordinary afternoon. When we got back to the Hotel, it was late, so we presumed the other people in our group already had plans for dinner. We decided to just have dinner alone at the hotel restaurant. It turned out to be a very good decision. The restaurant was not busy, the lights were subdued, just the proper ambiance for a quiet conversation. That was the first time, that we really talked about the time of my illness. I told Alberto how difficult it had been for me, not to be able to confide in him, for the first time in our married life. How I tried and hopefully succeeded in not letting him know how fearful and guilt-ridden I was. How I used to wonder, how he would adjust to a life alone. Of course, I knew the children would be there for him, to help him with the transition, but I knew it would be difficult for him. We had never been apart for long periods of time. I remembered a friend, who told me, when her husband died, that it was a good thing that they used to take separate vacations, I guess it sort of prepared her for the final separation. Well, Alberto and I never even thought of going on separate vacations. It just would be not be fun for either one of us. For his part, Alberto told me how badly he felt while he watched me suffer from the side effects of the chemotherapy and there was nothing he could do to share in it. So one day, he decided he would at least share in my prayers. That was when he asked me, if I wanted him to join me when I was praying the rosary and of course I said yes. It became our nightly ritual to pray the rosary together. He also told me he had tried to find out as much as he could about breast cancer, so he actually knew the statistics and it was silly of me to think that I was protecting him from knowing the facts, by not talking to him about it. We promised we would never keep secrets from each other again. We decided we would always share with each other whatever life may throw at us in the future. That was always the way we had done it in the past, from the time we first met and married in Pittsburgh and through the intervening years when we were happily raising our family. We never kept secrets from each other. We then talked about all those happy, carefree years before my illness. We reminisced over so many beautiful memories. And yet, I told Alberto that night, that as much as I cherished the "beautiful life" that we had enjoyed before my illness, at this time, in my mind, I had divided my life into the BC era ( before cancer) and AC era( after cancer) and I liked the AC era better. I feel it is much more balanced. When we finally left the restaurant to go up to our room, I thought what a perfect ending to an unusually blessed day!

Now that I am more aware of the presence of "moments rightly placed" in my life, I find that there are so many evidences of the unseen hand of God gently guiding me through life. There have been so many instances, when I have found to my amazement, answers to questions in my mind, in some unexpected events or places, proof that He not only guides me in important matters,but also in the small, seemingly inconsequential things in my life. I can only marvel at God's constant care for me. But of all the moments rightly placed in my life, the one that I am most grateful for was His bringing me to mass at the Monastery of the Blessed Sacrament, that morning, so I could get the message. If I had stayed home that morning as I had wanted to, if I had not been at mass to hear that homily, I might just have continued to feel very guilty, very hopeless, and I might not have been started on this spiritual journey, which has brought so much joy to my life. When I was first diagnosed with my illness, I knew I needed a miracle! I was begging God for the miracle of healing of the cancer, but now when I think of all that has happened in my life, I know that the greater miracle He gave me was my conversion journey, which has given me an awareness of His great mercy and love for me and His constant presence in my life. I can only hope and pray that this journey will continue for more years to come. I pray too, that as this journey continues, with the guidance of the Holy Spirit, I will gradually learn more and more to fully trust in God's will for me, and live each day accordingly. And whether this journey is a short or a long one I will always be very grateful. Every night, I pray, that when this journey comes to an end, as all journeys must, He will give me the courage and the wisdom, not to cling to the past, but with a heart full of joy and gratitude, fully accept His will to bring my journey to its end. I pray too, that He will give me the grace, to say, with my last breath, "I love You Lord; Your will be done."

## THE END